Have High Energy Every Day

**from the
Naturally Simple Health Series**

by

Stephanie Yeh

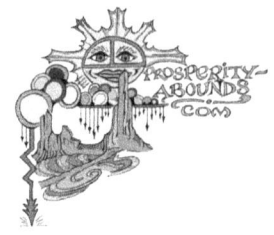

Contact Information: syeh@stephanieyeh.com
Visit my website: www.prosperity-abounds.com

Have High Energy Every Day
Easy Lifestyle Changes | Simple Habits

From the Naturally Simple Health Series

by Stephanie Yeh

Table of Contents

How to Have High Energy

√ Easy Lifestyle Changes
√ Simple Habits

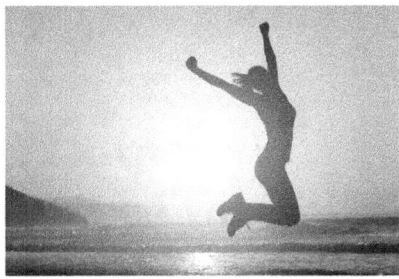

Expose Yourself (to Sunlight)! Getting just 10 to 15 minutes of exposure to sunlight can boost your circadian rhythm. This helps you feel more alert in the morning, and helps you power through an afternoon "slump."
(Columbia University Medical Center)

Fuel Your Tank and Jolt Your Brain. Waking up sluggish is normal—it's called 'sleep inertia'— because your body needs calories and your brain needs a wake-up call. Experts advise eating a breakfast with slow-release glucose, such as oatmeal and skim milk. Caffeine or supplements for the brain (ginseng, green tea, wheatgrass juice) can deliver the jolt your brain needs to emerge from the "brain fog."
(Tufts University)

Rock Out. Listening to upbeat music can help you access newfound energy when you feel tired or sluggish. Studies show that even thinking about this type of music can provide an energy boost. Experts note that how energetic you feel can be more about your *perception* of your level of energy than your *actual* energy level. Upbeat music can help you wake up more quickly in the morning, and help you dance through any period of sluggishness.
(University of Pittsburgh)

Have High Energy Every Day | **1** |

Have Low Energy?

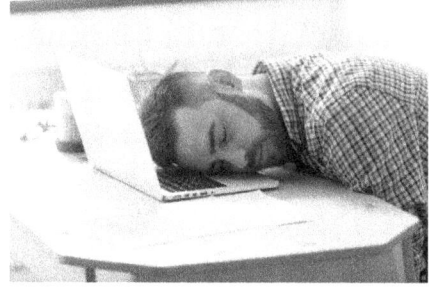

So do many Americans!

Did You Know That ...

- **Six out of seven people report waking up with low energy daily.**
  (Study by YouGov)

- **Fatigue is so common in U.S. workers that experts call it an epidemic.**
  (Journal of Occupational Medicine)

- **Despite feeling chronic fatigue, U.S. workers work an average of 47 hours per week.**
  (ohsonline)

- **Almost half of all Americans say they do not get enough sleep—and have enough energy—to safely do their jobs.**
  (National Safety Council)

- **97% of Americans have at least one of the top nine risk factors for fatigue and low energy.**
  (National Safety Council)

- **Low energy and job burnout can contribute to type 2 diabetes, coronary heart disease, high cholesterol, and even death for those 45 years or younger.**
  (Gallup)

Have High Energy Every Day | **2** |

High Energy: The Details

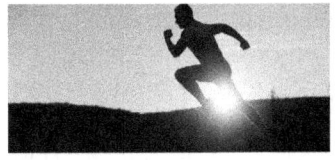

How much would your quality of life improve if you had high energy every single day? Whether it would help you feel better, work longer, or give you energy to enjoy your family, high energy is a big plus. The good news is that simple lifestyle hacks can boost your energy. Check out these uncommon tips...

Uncommon Tip #1: Chug Some Fluids

There are many contributors to feelings of fatigue. One of the most overlooked reasons for fatigue is simple dehydration. If you have consistently low energy at certain times of day drink more fluids before your energy slump. If you feel tired all the time, boost your fluid intake, especially early in the morning. Water, sports drinks, and juice are all good sources of fluids, with sports drinks and juice boosting your blood sugar as well as your hydration factor.

Uncommon Tip #2: Don't Give In to the Slump

When you feel low energy, the tendency is to take a nap or go to bed a few hours early. Unfortunately, while you may feel better in the short term, in the long term your body rhythms will be disturbed... and you will end up feeling more fatigued than ever. For higher energy, focus on going to bed and getting up at around the same time each day. Also, avoid snoozing on the couch in front of the television or napping after a heavy meal. Instead, take a walk or move around until bedtime.

Uncommon Tip #3: Breathe Deeply

Studies show that habitual shallow breathing can make you feel like you are in a "brain fog" or chronically tired, even if you get plenty of sleep. Meditation, yoga, and exercise can all help you breathe more deeply. Even a quick walk during your lunch break can help you feel much more energetic.

Have High Energy Every Day | **3** |

Uncommon Tip #4: Eat the Right Number of Calories

Feeling low energy is often the result of eating too few or too many calories. If you don't get enough calories daily, you will feel tired because you don't have enough fuel in your tank. You can also have low energy if you ingest too many calories because your system will go into overload and spend energy on digestion. To avoid either of these problems, women should get 1,600-2,400 calories daily, and men should get 2,000-3,000 calories every day (adjust for age, height, and weight).

(Office of Disease Prevention and Health Promotions)

Uncommon Tip #5: Get the Right Macronutrients in the Right Amount

Your brain and body both need all three macronutrients—carbohydrates, protein, and fats—to operate at a high level of energy. But these macronutrients need to be ingested in the right proportions. Some experts suggest 50% of calories from carbohydrates, 30% of calories from fat, and 20% of calories from protein.

Uncommon Tip #6: Check Your Magnesium Intake

While the main source of "fuel" for our cells is something called ATP (adenosine triphosphate), cells cannot actually make use of ATP unless the ATP is bound to a magnesium ion. In short, if your body lacks magnesium, your cells cannot get enough fuel to do their work. As a result you will feel low energy. Magnesium is also responsible for at least 300 enzymatic processes that keep your body and brain energized and healthy. To ensure that you get enough magnesium, eat foods rich in magnesium, such as spinach, pumpkin seeds, and almonds. You can also take a magnesium supplement. Consult your healthcare provider if you are unsure which source of magnesium would work best for you.

Get Your Free Consult for Having High Energy & Learn More about Healthy Lifestyles

Visit gohealth.tips/consult to get your free High Energy Consult from Prosperity-Abounds.

Common Sense Tips for High Energy

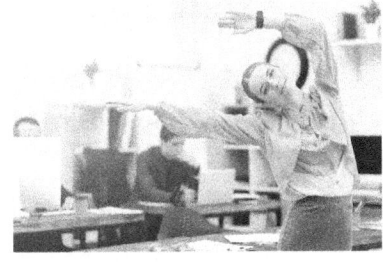

Want more simple and effective ways to have high energy all day long? Read the following common sense tips for better energy.

Common Sense Tip #1: Get Moving in the Afternoon

According to experts, our internal clocks make us prone to low energy between 2:00 pm and 4:00 pm. To counteract this natural energy dip, move your body during this time period. British researchers discovered that, regardless of the duration or intensity of the exercise, office workers who took exercise breaks felt more energetic, and showed a 15% improvement in job performance. (The Today Show)

Common Sense Tip #2: Eat Hearty Early, Eat Mini-Meals Later

Even though most people know the benefits of eating breakfast, studies show that a large percentage of U.S. workers consistently skip breakfast, choosing instead to drink coffee. But if you want a steady stream of high energy all morning long, eating a solid breakfast filled with complex carbs, protein, and a little fat will keep you going. To keep your blood sugar steady the rest of the day, eat smaller "mini" meals. Avoid eating a heavy lunch since that will result in a feeling of sluggishness during the afternoon.

Common Sense Tip #3: Start Strength Training

While engaging in any type of exercise is better than doing no exercise, studies show that strength training does the most to boost your energy. Strength training is any kind of movement that uses resistance to build muscle. Whether you use your own body weight, resistance bands, or weights to create resistance, strength training has been shown to raise physical energy levels more than other types of exercise. Of course, experts also suggest adding cardiovascular and flexibility training to any

strength training program. As with other types of movement meant to boost energy, any amount of strength training is better than none.
(National Institutes of Health)

Common Sense Tip #4: Add and Subtract from Your Diet

Eating the right kinds of food can really boost your energy levels daily. For instance, getting antioxidants from plant foods can help your body run more smoothly and efficiently. Cutting foods high in sugar and white flour will reduce inflammation in your body and boost energy. Finally, focus on foods high in omega-3 fatty acids, iron, vitamin B, zinc, magnesium, and vitamin D.

Common Sense Tip #5: Take Enzymes

One of the biggest causes of sluggish energy after a meal is poor digestion. While the food you eat and the resources in your body should allow you to fully digest what you eat, the sad truth is that your food and body often lack most of the enzymes you need for good digestion. The result is that your body has to work very hard to digest the food you eat without the help of extra enzymes. By taking enzymes (see gohealth.tips/digestion) with each meal, your body will be able to efficiently unlock the energy stored in the food you eat without expending a great deal of energy. The result? You get better energy throughout the day, and avoid the post meal slump!

Common Sense Tip #6: Set a Daily Meal Pattern

Many people who have difficulty eating healthy find that creating and sticking to a daily meal pattern can help create a steady

---

Supplements for High Energy Support

www.Prosperity-Abounds.com
1-866-384-4461 (toll free)

Enzymes (get the most energy from your food)
Get Enzymes at gohealth.tips/digestion

Whole Bluegreen Algae (bluegreen algae to fuel your **BODY**)
Get Whole Algae at gohealth.tips/AFA

Micro-blended Bluegreen Algae (bluegreen algae to clarify your **MIND**)
Get Micro-blended Algae at gohealth.tips/AFAMicro

High Energy Herbs & Nutrients (natural foods to boost energy)
Get High-Energy Supplements at gohealth.tips/energy

---

stream of high energy. By eating meals at the same time each day, your body won't go into starvation mood (which leads to low energy). Whether you choose to eat three meals a day, or two meals plus multiple mini-meals, just find a meal pattern that works for you. The only guideline is that most experts suggest avoiding a heavy meal close to the time you go to bed. Eating a heavy meal right before bed can lead to weight gain and sluggishness since the body does not digest well during sleep. Your body cannot get a full night's rest AND digest a large meal during the night.

Bonus Tips for High Energy

Need Some Quick Tips?

Desperate for better energy? Check out these overlooked tips for better energy:

- **If You Love Carbs, Add Some Fiber:** If you love eating carbohydrates, chances are that you feel an energy slump after you eat a high-carb meal. This happens because high carbs cause a high insulin response, which takes too much sugar out of your blood. Your brain then doesn't have enough fuel (sugars) to operate well, so it's hard to think clearly. By adding fiber into the mix, your body will slow digestion and the release of insulin. Voila! No after meal energy slump!

- **Snack Before You Sweat**: Many people find themselves skipping evening workouts because they feel too tired, even though exercise will boost their energy. If you have this problem, eat a quick snack before you sweat. Experts suggest eating about 250 calories with 25-35 grams of carbs, 10-15 grams of protein, and up to 5 grams of fat. A handful of pretzels or a healthy snack bar work well for this kind of snack.

- **Check Your Food Content:** If you feel that you eat healthy but still have low energy, check your food and liquid intake during the day. Be sure you eat at least two fruits or veggies during each meal, eat at least one fruit or veggie for each snack, and drink plenty of water during the day. Check with your healthcare provider for more specifics tailored to your level of health and height, weight, and body type.

- **Chew Some Gum:** If you need a quick energy boost, and you don't have time to eat a healthy meal or do some exercise, try chewing some gum. Some scientists believe that chewing gum improves energy and concentration because it increases circulation.

- **Blink More Often:** Research shows that staring at a computer screen for long periods can cause eye strain, leading to overall fatigue. To avoid this problem, look at something else while blinking for 20 seconds every 20 minutes. You will feel refreshed!

Feeling Young Again!

"For the last two decades of my software engineering career, I have been feeling very tired, and older than my actual age. When I had to stop swing dancing because I was too tired, I decided I needed to make a life change. I checked in with a local nutritionist and she helped me make great lifestyle changes. In addition to eating a healthier diet, I started a yoga class, and started taking a couple of short walks during the work day. Certain supplements (CoQ10, bluegreen algae, and herbs for mental clarity) also gave me a huge energy boost. I feel younger than I have in years!"

~ Sue Erlichman, Holland, MI

High Energy Success Profile

Profile: Fred Wilson, age 62

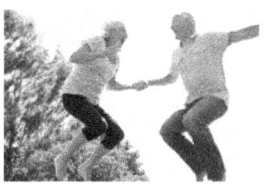

Goal: Have enough daily energy for a busy and active lifestyle

Strategy for Success: After doing his own research, Fred decided to use the following strategies to boost his daily energy:

- **Hydrate and Snack:** Using an online water intake calculator, Fred realized that he was not drinking the recommended amount of water based on his weight and age—about 10.5 cups of water. To stay hydrated Fred drank as much water as possible early in the day, and also before and after workouts. Fred also added a couple of snacks to his meal pattern—one before working out, and one before his afternoon slump.

- **Add Macro and Micronutrients:** Fred started eating more balanced meals with the right amounts of carbs, fat, and protein. In addition, Fred began taking bluegreen algae, magnesium, CoQ10 (gohealth.tips/coq10), enzymes (gohealth.tips/digestion), and other pre-packaged supplements (gohealth.tips/daily) filled with ingredients to boost mental clarity and physical energy.

- **Eat More Fiber:** With a love of carbohydrates, Fred was thrilled that he did not need to give up carbs altogether. Instead he focused on adding fiber to his diet, both from whole foods (fruits and veggies) and with a fiber supplement recommended by his doctor.

- **Get Sun:** To combat sleepiness in the morning and after lunch, Fred started getting sun exposure early in the morning and an hour or two after lunch.

Results: With just a few tweaks to his daily habits, Fred was able to gain a great deal more daily energy. Not only does Fred work a full-time job, but he has enough energy to workout at the gym three times a week, cycle on the weekends, and participate in an active social life. Needless to say, Fred is thrilled!

Frequently Asked Questions About Having High Energy

If I want to eat snacks that will boost my energy, what are the best snacks to eat?

Experts suggest eating foods with a "low glycemic index," which means foods with sugar content that break down at a slow rate. Most whole foods such as fruits, vegetables, and nuts have this property. The best fruits to eat include grapes, apples, bananas, oranges, peaches, and grapefruit. Leafy greens are the best vegetables to eat. Peas and beans are also whole foods with a low glycemic index. Most nuts provide plenty of protein, fiber, and fat, and experts favor almonds, peanuts, brazil nuts, pine nuts, pecans, pistachios, and walnuts.

What should I eat if I want to recover from illness and regain my energy levels quickly?

While whole vegetables are great to provide the necessary nutrients to help with illness recovery, if you are already sick your body often does not have enough energy to digest the fiber in the vegetables. One way to get the maximum nutrients from vegetables without forcing your body to work hard at digestion is to drink juiced vegetables. With all the antioxidants, vitamins, minerals, and nutrients in vegetable juice, your body has easy access to the building blocks to boost energy and support immunity to help you recover more quickly. Stay away from store-bought juices that are high in sugar or unpronounceable additives. Stick with juices that list vegetable juice as the main ingredients, with as few additives as possible. Sugary juices will leave you feeling worse, not better.

How do sleep habits impact energy levels, and what can I do to improve my sleep?

The amount of <u>satisfactory</u> sleep that you get each night plays a huge role in the amount of energy you have. Regardless of the amount of time you sleep in bed, if you don't get enough sleep that satisfies your body and mind, you will still wake up tired. Good sleep is often dependent on your body's ability to successfully cycle through the phases of REM and non-REM sleep. To improve sleep, stick to a sleep schedule, and avoid napping or going to bed early even when you are tired. Experts also suggest limiting alcohol and sugar intake, getting exposure to sunlight morning and afternoon, and making exercise a regular part of your life.

Why do experts recommend exercising for higher energy? I am usually so tired that the thought of exercise makes me tired.

Many people with low energy struggle with the catch-22 of tiredness and exercise. Experts recommend exercise as a solution to low energy, but when you feel tired, the last thing you feel like doing is suiting up for a sweat session. But if you can get over the "hump" and force yourself to start moving, you <u>will</u> feel more energetic. Exercise gets the blood moving and releases substances like endorphins and adrenaline, which will raise your energy levels and reduce sensations of pain and fatigue. Get this: experts say that we don't "get" energy, we create energy. Simply moving your body—even with a few jumping jacks or strength exercises—will actually "charge up" your cells. The result? You feel more alive, energetic, and happier (since many mood neurotransmitters are released during exercise). So even if you are tired at the end of your work day or at the start of your day, take 15 minutes to exercise. You will be amazed at the change in your energy levels!

Are there other options to exercise to boost energy?

If stress and tension are the main causes of your low energy, practices such as yoga or meditation can boost your energy levels through relaxation and a sense of calm. Studies show that people who participate in just 25 minutes of yoga get a significant energy boost, which contributes to good mood. Even better, studies show that relaxation techniques actually strengthen the immune system, and allow people to be more resilient in the face of stressful situations.

Resources for Having High Energy

Specific supplements can be helpful when you want to boost your energy levels. Some of the most highly recommended supplements for energy support include:

- **Vitamin D**: The body makes this vitamin when skin is exposed to the sun. This vitamin regulates insulin secretion and metabolism, both of which can strongly affect energy levels. With insufficient vitamin D, the body can secrete too much insulin, robbing the blood of too many sugars, leaving the brain and body short of "fuel." In addition, vitamin D, gained through sun exposure, can help boost energy, especially in the morning and in the early afternoon. This helps avoid morning "brain fog" and the after lunch "slump"!

- **Vitamin B12**: This vitamin is necessary for almost every bodily function and for energy production. Vitamin B12 is needed to create new red blood cells, maintain the function of the nervous system, and support the heart, bones, and brain. If you are low in B12, you can feel tired, moody, and irritable. The best sources of B12, aside from a supplement, are shellfish, red meat, eggs, clams, and fortified cereal grains.

- **CoEnzyme Q10**: This enzyme is key to your cells being able to produce usable energy. As the body ages, its ability to generate CoQ10 decreases, so taking a CoQ10 supplement can have a strong positive effect on physical energy levels (see gohealth.tips/coq10).

- **Ashwaganda**: This adaptogenic herb has a strong influence on the body's adrenal function and energy levels. When the adrenal glands are overworked, the results include low energy, moodiness, and hormonal and endocrine issues. This herb regulates cortisol (the stress hormone), supports the adrenals, improves endurance, and increases overall energy.

- **Ginseng**: Both American and Asian ginseng have been used to provide increased energy, reduce stress and anxiety, and stabilize mood. Because not all ginseng is of the same quality, be sure to purchase from a reputable source. Also consult your healthcare provider before taking this herb to avoid side effects or possible drug interactions.

- **Rhodiala Rosea**: This herb is known for its energy enhancing and brain boosting powers. Rhodiala can help your brain and body adapt to environmental and chemical stress. This herb also can help balance the stress hormone cortisol, which in turn supports better energy production in the body.

- **AFA Bluegreen Algae**: This tiny wholefood supplement provides a full spectrum of micro and macronutrients that the body can use to produce energy, clean the body of toxins, and support the brain. When added to other herbs, enzymes or probiotics (see gohealth.tips/digestion), this form of blugreen algae (whole cell for physical energy in the BODY or micro-blended for mental clarity for the MIND) can provide a huge boost for your body's energy production. Learn more at www.prosperity-abounds.com.

Get Your Free Consult on Having High Energy & Learn More about Healthy Lifestyles

Visit gohealth.tips/consult to get your free High Energy Consult from Prosperity-Abounds.

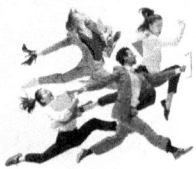

www.Prosperity-Abounds.com | 1-866-384-4461 (toll free)

High Energy Hacks from Real People

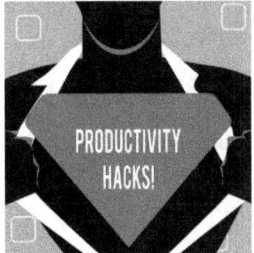

One of the best ways to have high energy all day is to learn from people who have figured out tips and tricks for gaining and maintaining high energy. Read through the wide variety of high energy hacks from real people, and pick out the ones that match your lifestyle and desired energy level!

Have an "Anything Goes" Day

"A long time ago I realized the power of having one day a week to recharge my batteries. I call this my 'Anything Goes' day. While the day of the week I choose for recharging my energy may change, my rules about this day never do. The rules are simple. One, unless there is a major emergency, having this day to myself is non-negotiable. Two, I never plan a schedule on my recharge day so that I can be free to do whatever I feel like... or nothing at all. Three, I let myself sleep, eat, drink, and entertain myself however I like (no diets, no alarm clocks). Sometimes I spend the day in my PJs and binge-watching episodes of my favorite shows, On other recharge days I'm actually very productive. The point is that giving myself complete freedom on these special days never fails to recharge my energy for the week ahead. Plus, when I have a rough week, I get to look forward to my 'Anything Goes' day!"
~ Melissa D., Montgomery, AL

Tap the Thymus

"This is a very cool trick I learned from my acupuncturist to boost my energy. She showed me how to use two fingers to slowly and gently tap my sternum (the thymus is behind the sternum) about 30 times while breathing deeply. I can truly say that this seems to tell my body to wake up and get energized. I do this anytime I feel tired, sometimes as much as 10 times a day."
~ Tara H., Wellford, SC

Have High Energy Every Day | **19** |

Avoid Energy Vampires

"I used to think people were nuts when they talked about energy vampires until a transfer student moved into our college dorm. Wow! Every time I was around this person I felt like I needed to take a nap or drink a gallon of coffee. I can't tell you what this person did that made it so tiring to hang out with him, but his effect on me (and other people in our dorm) was unmistakable. Needless to say I avoided this person as much as possible. Since college I have met more people who fall into the 'energy vampire' category. When I meet these kinds of people I run in the other direction. I make it a conscious effort to surround myself with people who energize me. It makes a huge difference to my daily energy."
~ Jonah S., Port Madison, WA

Swallow Some Sunshine

"It is no secret that exposure to sunshine helps awaken the body and mind. If you feel sluggish or tired, and you cannot go stand in the sunshine for 15 minutes, another option is to swallow some sunshine. As a nutritionist, I often suggest people take AFA bluegreen algae supplements because taking algae offers some of the same benefits as sunshine (see gohealth.tips/AFA). This type of algae uses photosynthesis to convert sunlight to amino acids and numerous nutrients the body can use. In fact, this type of algae has a nutritional profile that is very close to mother's milk."
~ Allison L., Cincinnati, OH

Snack on Energy-Rich Foods

"As a fitness trainer I always check that my clients have fuel in the tank before each workout. While it is not a good idea to eat a heavy meal before a workout, eating a healthy snack rich in healthy nutrients can mean the difference between a productive fitness session and a torturous one. I often suggest my clients eat a healthy snack bar or a handful of nuts as a great way to fuel the body before exercise."
~ Betsy U., Nashville, TN

Have High Energy Every Day | **20** |

Take Care of That Nagging Feeling

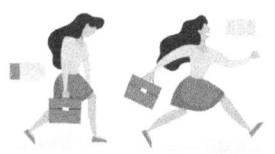
"Do you ever get a nagging feeling about a task you need to do or a conversation you need to have? Regardless of whether the task or conversation or whatever is truly urgent or not, the nagging feeling that goes with it can be a big energy drain. I've learned that taking just 15 minutes to clear that item off my desk can free up my mind and boost my energy. Most of the time the item is NOT urgent, but the need to get rid of the nagging feeling IS urgent. This little trick has saved me from many a non-productive day."
~ Tricia C., Aurora, CO

Do the Sit-Stand-Sit Routine

"As a writer I spend a lot of time sitting in front of my computer. I can get so wrapped up in what I am doing that hours can fly by before I get up for a break. But to be honest, my productivity goes down the longer I sit in front of my computer. Plus, I get really tired. My chiropractor suggested I buy a tabletop stand for my laptop, and switch between sitting and standing while I work on the computer. Apparently, studies show that changing positions keeps the brain and body more alert and focused. Since I've been using this technique, I find that my body doesn't get nearly as fatigued, and my brain seems more productive and energetic."
~ Adam E., Philadelphia, PA

Swallow Essential Nutrients Before a Slump

"Almost everyone I know is prone to an energy 'slump' at a certain part of the day. Mine is either mid-morning or early afternoon. I used to reach for chips or crackers whenever I experienced an energy slump, but I found that the energy I got from these snacks did not last very long. A friend suggested I try taking nutrients in a more direct form—something that does not require digestion. I started taking convenient nutritional packets that included AFA bluegreen algae, probiotics, and enzymes (see gohealth.tips/daily). When taken *before* my energy slump, these

packets keep my energy humming along at a steady pace all day long."
~ Don K., Houston, TX

Take a Hot and Cold Shower
"When I took a gap year between high school and college, I was fortunate to be able to travel to several countries outside the U.S. I have always heard about the value of a hot shower to ease aches and cold showers to wake up. In my travels I discovered that some cultures use alternating hot and cold water showers (going between hot and cold water several times per shower) to energize the body for the day. I have used this technique for years to wake up, stay awake, and keep my energy high. This is a super simple way to get high energy, and has since been proven effective by scientific studies."
~ Olivia G., Fairfield Glade, TN

Smell Something Good
"Of the five senses, did you know that the sense of smell has the most direct route to the brain? It is the reason that the smell of chocolate chip cookies is so comforting. By the same token, taking a whiff of cinnamon or spearmint can energize your body and help you feel more alert. When I work long hours, I use aromatherapy to keep my energy high and my brain clear."
~ John W., Cape May, NJ

Exercise Before a Long Day
"My best friend is a personal trainer and she knows a lot about sports medicine and psychology. One day I was complaining to her, as usual, about my long hours and fatigue, and she sort of read me the riot act. She was constantly trying to get me to go to the gym after work, but I was always running on empty at the end of the day. My friend finally lost her patience and made me a bet. She bet me $200 that she could create an exercise program that would not only fit into my day, but would give me enough energy, after 30 days, to help survive my job. I took the bet because I was sure I was going to earn a quick $200! What I didn't know was that my friend was going to show up at my front door every morning at 5:00 am with a smile and coffee. She

dragged me through a short workout every morning that nevertheless had me panting and sweating after just 10 minutes. The first week I thought I was going to win the bet because I was more tired than ever. That's why I was so surprised that I felt amazingly energetic at the end of the bet. I still didn't like getting up so early to work out, but I loved having enough energy to make it all the way through the day! Believe me when I say that losing the bet was the best $200 I ever spent! My friend later explained that exercise not only generates 'feel good' neurotransmitters (think runner's high), but also sets up the body and mind to feel energized and happy for the rest of the day."
~ Catherine F., Milwaukee, WI

Organize or Clean

"My friends have always joked that they can tell how I feel by the state of my house. When things are piled up everywhere or my kitchen floor is sticky, my friends know I don't feel very energetic or excited about life. I discovered that I could use the relationship between my energy level and the state of my house to boost my energy. What I mean is this: whenever I feel depressed by all the piles of clutter around my house, I can quickly boost my energy by organizing and cleaning my house. I feel instantly better when I look at a room I have just cleaned and organized. Some self-help books suggest doing the same at work—tidying up your desk so you feel clear and energized about your work!"
~ Elizabeth M., Atlanta, GA

Change Something to Avoid Getting Stuck in a Rut

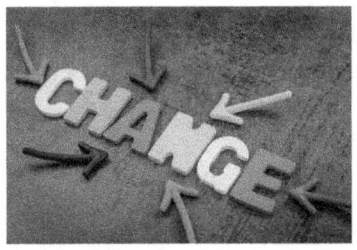

"One of my favorite sayings is, 'A grave is only a few feet deeper than a rut, so don't get stuck in a rut!' I know I'm stuck in a rut when I feel tired and bored with my life. Luckily I am a big fan of change. Sometimes I move my furniture around to give my house a new look. Other times, I change little things, such as which hand I use to open a door. The possibilities for change are endless, from trying out a new restaurant for lunch to picking a different route

or time to get to work. Every time I make this kind of change I get a boost of energy because change makes my life feel new and fresh."
~ Paulina V., Scottsdale, AZ

Try Dry Brushing
"If you need an energy boost but don't have time for a full workout or a full night's sleep, try dry brushing. As a bodywork therapist, I offer all kinds of services to rejuvenate the body. Dry brushing, which is nothing more than lightly buffing the skin with a dry natural-bristle brush, is one of my favorites. More than one of my clients has reported feeling energized and more 'alive' after a dry brushing session (which can take as little as 15 minutes). The great thing about dry brushing is that you can buy a long-handled brush and dry brush your whole body. Not only does this technique get your circulation moving, but your skin also looks and feels great."
~ Grayson T., Newark, DE

Tackle the Tough Stuff
"Nothing drags me down as fast as a 'yucky' task that I am avoiding. A business coach taught me how to stop avoiding tough tasks, and to tackle them first. This way I get the difficult part of my day done first, making the rest of the day a nice down hill slide. I am always amazed at how happy and energetic I feel when I complete that difficult job. These days tackling the tough stuff first has become habit, so I actually look forward to sinking my teeth into a tough task!"
~ Mary H., Manchester, NH

Get Your Free
High Energy Consult

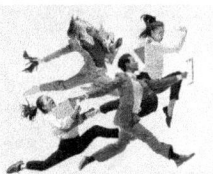

About the Author

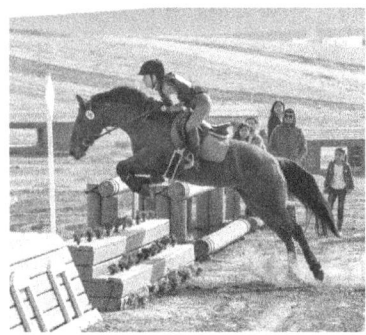

Stephanie Yeh has been researching, learning, and publishing about natural health solutions for over 20 years. Her interests include the use of whole foods, natural supplements, herbs, flower essences, homeopathics, vibrational healing, Edgar Cayce remedies, and bodywork for people and animals.

She has partnered with a wide variety of people to create vibrant natural health for people and their pets.

Stephanie is super passionate about horses and their health, and has enjoyed helping many rescued equines regain health and happiness.

Stephanie enjoys sharing her knowledge of natural healing through a variety of channels, including:

Website: www.Prosperity-Abounds.com

Blog: Prosperity-Abounds.Blogspot.com

Nutritional Consultations: gohealth.tips/consult

Have High Energy Every Day | **26** |

.

www.ingramcontent.com/pod-product-compliance
Lightning Source LLC
Chambersburg PA
CBHW070258290526
45791CB00011B/1624